36 Delicious Low Carb Slow Cooker Paleo Chicken Recipes

Paleo Chicken Recipes For Weight Loss

BY

MONICA MARIE

I0435505

What is paleo and what does it consist of?

The paleo diet consists of the solely consumption of meat, nuts, vegetables, fruits, plants and water. Research shows that paleo diet is one of the most effective lifestyles for fat loss and overall health. It can prevent diseases that are overwhelming within the current population and add high levels of energy into someone's daily routine. Paleo is a lifetime way of eating, when you follow a paleo diet you try to eat as similar as possible to our generic heritage from the previous millenniums, those that were hunters and gatherers and did not have the means or the technology to consume the types of processed foods that exist today.

How will these recipes help me?

If you take a quick look into the past, you will see that our ancestors were physically big and strong. They did not know or suffered from any of the many incurable diseases that society faces today such as cancer, diabetes, polio, etc. The change in nutrition has had a huge impact on this, we have moved from eating plants and animals to eating products filled with refined grains and sugar. For this reason, some of the most recognized health experts recommend the paleo diet as a way to enhance our lives and live in a more healthy and energetic way.

What types of food will I be able to eat?

The following model describes the paleo diet best, if it doesn't fly, swim, walks or doesn't grow on the ground, don't eat it. When you follow the paleo diet you need to mainly consume the following foods: beef, poultry, eggs, nuts, fruits, seeds and fibrous vegetables, in other words, **one ingredient foods**. In the paleo diet, foods such as candy, bread, chips, cookies, processed juices should not be allowed. Many types of grains and diary should also not be consumed if you want to properly follow and reap the health benefits of this powerful diet.

What will I get from this eBook?

In this book I have included **36 easy to make, delicious low carb paleo chicken recipes** that will get you started in the journey to transforming your health and body. These recipes are easy to make and can be cooked in any occasion. I hope you love making these recipes as much as I do. Enjoy!

Chicken and Sweet Potato Stew
Serves 4

Ingredients:

- 1 pound boneless, skinless chicken breasts
- 1 yellow onion, diced
- 3 carrots, peeled and diced
- 1 large sweet potato, peeled and diced
- 4 cloves of garlic, minced
- 2 cups homemade chicken broth
- 1 can tomato paste
- 3 tablespoons balsamic vinegar
- 2 teaspoons whole grain mustard
- 2 bay leaves
- 2 cups baby spinach
- Sea salt and pepper to taste

Instructions:

1. Cut chicken breasts into chunks and add to the pot of your slow cooker.
2. Add the onion, carrots, sweet potato, garlic, chicken broth, tomato paste, balsamic vinegar, mustard, and bay leaves. Stir to combine. Season with salt and pepper.
3. Place slow cooker on high for 4-5 hours or low for 6-8 hours.
4. An hour before serving, add the spinach and mix well.
5. Serve and enjoy! Store any leftovers in an airtight container in the refrigerator or freezer.

Ginger & Apple Shredded Chicken
Serves 6-8

Ingredients:

- 2 pounds boneless, skinless chicken breasts
- 1 yellow onion, sliced
- 2 apples, cored and sliced (Granny Smith's work great)
- 1 cup chicken broth or water
- 2 tablespoons freshly grated ginger
- 1 tablespoon honey
- 1 teaspoon cinnamon
- ½ teaspoon smoked paprika
- 1 teaspoon salt
- ½ teaspoon black pepper
- 2 cloves of garlic, minced
- 1 bay leaf

Instructions:

1. Pour the chicken broth or water into your slow cooker.
2. Layer the onions, chicken and apples into the slow cooker.
3. Add the spices, ginger, and honey.
4. Cook for 8-10 hours on low or 6-8 hours on high.
5. Use tongs or two forks to shred the chicken once it'd done cooking.
6. Serve!

Chicken Enchilada Stew
Serves 6-8

Ingredients:

- 2 pounds boneless, skinless chicken breasts
- 1 green bell pepper, diced
- 1 yellow onion, diced
- 1 (4 ounce) can chopped green chilies
- 1 (4 ounce) can chopped jalapenos
- 2 tablespoons olive oil
- 1 (14 ounce) can diced tomatoes
- 1 (7 ounce) can tomato sauce
- 4 cloves of garlic, minced
- 1 tablespoon chili powder
- 1 tablespoon cumin
- 2 teaspoons oregano
- sea salt and pepper to taste
- Avocado, diced (garnish)
- Cilantro, chopped (garnish)

Instructions:

1. Place chicken breasts in your slow cooker.
2. Sprinkle the spices on top then add the remainder of the ingredients (except for the garnishes).
3. Cook on low for 8-10 hours or high for 6-8 hours.
4. When it's done cooking, use tongs or two forks to shred the chicken apart and mix well with the other ingredients.
5. Top with avocado and cilantro. Enjoy!

Spicy Pulled Chicken Chili
Serves 6-8

Ingredients:

- 2 pounds boneless chicken breasts and/or thighs
- 2 yellow onions, diced
- 2 bell peppers, diced
- 2 (14 ounce) cans fire roasted tomatoes
- 1 (14 ounce) can tomato sauce
- 3 cloves of garlic, peeled
- ½ cup hot sauce of your choice (or omit for less spiciness)
- 3 tablespoons smoked paprika
- 2 tablespoons garlic powder
- 1 tablespoon red pepper flakes
- 1 tablespoon cumin
- sea salt and pepper to taste
- Green onions, sliced (garnish)
- Avocado, diced (garnish)

Instructions:

1. Place chicken breasts/thighs in your slow cooker.
2. Make three small cuts into the chicken and stuff the garlic cloves in.
3. Pour the hot sauce over the chicken.
4. Sprinkle with all of the spices.
5. Place the onions, bell peppers, roasted tomatoes, and tomato sauce over the top.
6. Cook on low for 8-10 hours or high for 6-8 hours.
7. Top with sliced green onions and avocado before serving.

Spicy Mustard Slow Cooker Chicken
Serves 2

Ingredients

- 2 Chicken Breasts
- 1/2 Red Bell Pepper, sliced
- 1/2 Green Bell Pepper, sliced
- 3-4 Carrots, sliced
- 3-4 Celery Stalks, sliced
- 2/3 cup Chicken Broth
- 2-3 TBSP Olive Oil
- 2 TBSP Garlic Chili Sauce
- 2 TBSP Honey
- 3 TBSP Dijon Mustard
- 2 tsp Onion Powder
- 2 tsp Black Pepper
- 2 TBSP Ground Mustard Powder

Instructions

1. Place the chicken breasts in your slow cooker, evenly spread out
2. In a mix bowl, combine the Chicken Broth, Olive Oil, Garlic Chili Sauce, Honey, Dijon Mustard, Onion Powder, Black Pepper & Ground Mustard Powder. Stir until fully mixed.
3. Pour the sauce mixture over the Chicken Breasts in your slow cooker
4. Put the lid on and set on LOW for 3 1/2 hours
5. After 2 hours, add the Celery, Carrots, Bell Peppers, put the lid back on and let cook for the remaining 1 1/2 hours
6. If it's a workout day and you're having rice, prepare according the instructions on the bag (omit the rice for a great "anytime" meal)
7. Place the chicken, vegetables and sauce over the rice and enjoy your awesomeness in the kitchen!

Chicken Chili Verde
Serves 5-6

Ingredients:

- 2 pounds boneless chicken breasts and/or thighs
- 2 jalapeno peppers, deseeded and cut in half
- 2 poblano peppers, deseeded and cut in half
- 8-10 tomatillos, husked and cut in half
- 2 tablespoons olive oil
- 1 small onion, diced
- 2 cloves of garlic, minced
- ½ cup lime juice
- 2 teaspoons oregano
- 1 teaspoon cumin
- sea salt and pepper to taste
- 2 cups chicken broth or water

Instructions:

1. Preheat oven to 450 degrees Fahrenheit.
2. Place the jalapenos, poblanos, and tomatillos on a metal baking sheet and drizzle with the olive oil. Cook for 20-30 minutes, until charred on the outside. Allow to cook and run the peppers under cool water to remove the charred skin.
3. In a food processor or blender, pulse the cooked peppers and tomatillos with the onion, garlic, and lime juice until well combined.
4. Place the chicken in your slow cooker, cover with the pepper/tomatillo puree, and sprinkle with spices.
5. Pour the broth over everything and cook on low for 8 hours.
6. Garnish with lime wedges and cilantro, if desired.

Coconut Curry Chicken
Serves 6-8

Ingredients:

- 3 pounds boneless chicken breasts and/or thighs
- 1 yellow onion, diced
- 2 carrots, peeled and diced
- 2 cloves of garlic, minced
- 1 tablespoon curry powder
- 2 teaspoons turmeric
- 1 teaspoon sea salt
- 1 teaspoon pepper
- 1 tablespoon yellow mustard
- ½ cup coconut milk (canned)
- ½ cup chicken stock
- 2 tablespoons coconut oil, melted

Instructions:

1. Place the onion, carrots, and garlic in the bottom of your slow cooker.
2. Layer the chicken on top of the vegetables and sprinkle the spices on.
3. Whisk together the melted coconut oil, coconut milk, and chicken broth. Pour over the chicken.
4. Cook on low for 6-8 hours.
5. When done cooking, remove the chicken from the slow cooker and puree the sauce with an immersion blender.
6. Pour the sauce over the chicken and serve immediately.

Smoky-Sweet Pulled Chicken
Serves 4-6

Ingredients:

- 2 ½ pounds boneless, skinless chicken breasts and thighs
- 4 cloves of garlic
- 1 tablespoon smoked paprika
- 1-2 chipotle peppers in adobo sauce (depending on desired spiciness)
- ½ cup pomegranate seeds
- 2 teaspoons sea salt

Instructions:

1. Place chicken in the bottom of your slow cooker.
2. Sprinkle the salt and smoked paprika over the chicken.
3. Make 4 small cuts in the chicken and tuck the garlic cloves into them.
4. Finely dice the chipotle pepper(s) and add to the slow cooker.
5. Cook on low for 8-9 hours.
6. Once finished cooking, use tongs or two forks to shred the chicken.
7. Stir in the pomegranate seeds and serve. Makes a great addition to tacos, salads, etc.

Jerk Chicken Legs
Serves 4

Ingredients:

- 4 (each) chicken drumsticks and wings
- 4 teaspoons paprika
- 4 teaspoons sea salt
- 2 teaspoons garlic powder
- 2 teaspoons white pepper
- 2 teaspoons thyme
- 2 teaspoons onion powder
- 1 teaspoon cayenne pepper

Instructions:

1. Mix all of the spices together in a small bowl.
2. Pat the chicken dry and rub the spice mixture over the meat thoroughly, trying to get it under the skin, if possible.
3. Place the chicken in your slow cooker and cook on low for 5-6 hours.
4. Chicken will easily fall from the bone once done.

Honey-Dijon Whole Roasted Chicken
Serves 4-6

Ingredients:

- 1 whole chicken, about 3 pounds (make sure it'll fit in your slow cooker)
- 1 lemon, zested and juiced
- ¼ cup honey
- 2 tablespoons Dijon mustard
- ½ white onion, quartered
- 3 cloves of garlic, peeled
- 3 sprigs of rosemary
- sea salt and pepper to taste

Instructions:

1. Remove the giblets and pat your chicken dry.
2. Season generously with salt and pepper and place in the slow cooker.
3. Finely chop the rosemary and combine with the lemon juice, lemon zest, honey, and mustard. Mix well and brush all over the chicken, using all of the mixture.
4. Place the garlic, quartered onion, and lemon halves inside of the chicken.
5. Cook on low for 6 hours.
6. Serve and enjoy!

Brazilian Curried Chicken
Serves 4-5

Ingredients:

- 2 pounds boneless, skinless chicken breasts and thighs
- 1 cup coconut milk (canned)
- 2 tablespoons tomato paste
- 3 cloves of garlic, minced
- 4 tablespoons curry powder
- 1 tablespoon ground ginger
- 1 yellow onion, thinly sliced
- 2 bell peppers, thinly sliced
- sea salt and pepper to taste
- 1 cup chicken stock

Instructions:

1. In your slow cooker, whisk together the coconut milk, tomato paste, garlic, ginger, curry powder, salt, and pepper.
2. Add the sliced onion and peppers.
3. Layer the chicken on top and pour the broth over everything.
4. Cook on low for 6-8 hours or high for 4-5 hours.
5. Done! Try serving it over cauliflower "rice" or spaghetti squash.

Chicken Stuffed Peppers
Serves 4

Ingredients:

- 4 bell peppers (any color)
- 1 pound ground chicken
- ½ head cauliflower
- 1 yellow onion, diced
- 2 carrots, peeled and diced
- 4 cloves of garlic, minced
- 1 (6 ounce) can tomato paste
- 3 tablespoons Italian seasoning
- ¼ cup beef stock
- sea salt and pepper to taste

Instructions:

1. Place the cauliflower, onion, carrots, and garlic in a food processor. Pulse until finely ground.
2. Cut the tops off of your peppers and remove the seeds.
3. Mix the vegetables with the ground chicken, and tomato paste. Season with Italian seasoning and salt and pepper.
4. Spoon the mixture into the peppers and place in your slow cooker. Make sure to place the pepper tops back on.
5. Pour the beef stock in the bottom of the slow cooker and cook for 6-8 hours on low.
6. Enjoy!

Fire Roasted Chicken Chili
Serves 4

Ingredients:

- 1 pound boneless, skinless chicken breasts
- 3 bell peppers (any color), diced
- 1 red onion, diced
- 1 jalapeno, deseeded and diced
- 2 cloves of garlic, minced
- 2 cups salsa
- 1 ½ cup water
- 1 teaspoon cumin
- 2 teaspoons chili powder
- Sea salt and pepper to taste
- 1 avocado, diced

Instructions:

1. Place chicken breasts in the bottom of your slow cooker.
2. Sprinkle with the cumin, chili powder, and salt and pepper.
3. Add the salsa and diced onion. Cook on low for 6-8 hours.
4. Once the chicken is done cooking, shred with tongs or two forks.
5. Sauté the bell peppers and jalapeno over medium-high heat, until well roasted.
6. Add the peppers to the slow cooker and stir to mix well.
7. Add the water to slow cooker and cook for an additional 20 minutes.
8. Top with avocado before serving.

Acorn Squash Soup
Serves 4-6

Ingredients:

- 1 pound ground chicken
- 1 acorn squash, peeled and diced into medium sized cubes
- 1 tablespoon coconut oil
- 4 cups chicken stock
- 4 cups water
- 1 red onion, diced
- 2 cloves of garlic, minced
- 2 teaspoons dried parsley
- Sea salt and pepper to taste

Instructions:

1. Add the coconut oil to a large skillet and cook the chicken until browned.
2. Place the squash, onion, garlic, and seasonings to your slow cooker.
3. Add the ground chicken and deglaze the pan with 1 cup of chicken stock. Add to the slow cooker.
4. Pour in the remaining liquid and cook on low for 4-6 hours.
5. Serve and enjoy!

Cashew Chicken
Serves 4-6

Ingredients:

- 2 pounds boneless boneless chicken thighs, cut into 1" pieces
- ¼ cup arrowroot powder
- 1 teaspoon black pepper
- 1 tablespoon coconut oil
- 3 tablespoons coconut aminos
- 2 tablespoons rice wine vinegar
- 2 tablespoons tomato paste
- 2 cloves of garlic, minced
- 1 teaspoon ginger, minced
- 1 teaspoon crushed red pepper
- ½ cup raw cashews

Instructions:

1. Place the arrowroot powder and black pepper in a large zip top bag. Add the chicken pieces and shake to thoroughly coat.
2. Melt the coconut oil in a large skillet over medium-high heat. Cook the chicken until browned on all sides. Add to your slow cooker.
3. Mix together the coconut aminos, vinegar, tomato paste, garlic, ginger, and crushed red pepper in a small bowl. Pour over the chicken.
4. Cook on low for 4-5 hours.
5. Stir in the raw cashews just before serving.

Moroccan Chicken and Sweet Potatoes
Serves 4-6

Ingredients:

- 2 pounds chicken thighs and drumsticks
- 1 tablespoon coconut oil
- ½ yellow onion, sliced
- 1 teaspoon cumin
- 1 teaspoon turmeric
- 1 teaspoon cinnamon
- ½ teaspoon cardamom
- ½ teaspoon chili powder
- ½ teaspoon coriander
- 4 cloves of garlic
- 2 tablespoons fresh ginger, grated
- 2 cups chicken stock
- 1 cup dried apricots
- 2 cups sweet potatoes, diced

Instructions:

1. Combine the spices and minced garlic in a small bowl.
2. In a large skillet over medium-high heat, melt the coconut oil. Cook the chicken until browned on all sides. Transfer to your slow cooker.
3. Add the onions to the pan and sauté for 3-4 minutes. Add the spice mixture and cook for another minute.
4. Remove from heat and stir in the stock and grated ginger. Pour over the chicken.
5. Cook on low for 3 hours.
6. Add the dried apricots and sweet potatoes and cook for another 3 hours on low.
7. Garnish with fresh cilantro, if desired.

Pineapple Pulled Chicken
Serves 6-8

Ingredients:

- 2 pounds boneless, skinless chicken breasts
- 2 cups pineapple, diced
- 4 cloves of garlic
- 1 yellow onion, sliced
- 1 red bell pepper, sliced
- ½ cup chicken stock
- juice of 1 lemon
- juice of 1 lime
- 1 teaspoon chili powder
- Sea salt and pepper to taste
- Green onions, sliced (garnish)

Instructions:

1. Add all ingredients to your slow cooker except for the pineapple and green onions.
2. Place the pineapple on top of everything.
3. Cook on low for 6-8 hours.
4. When done cooking, shred the chicken with tongs or two forks.
5. Garnish with sliced green onions and serve.

Chicken Cacciatore
Serves 6

Ingredients:

- 2 white onions, minced
- ¼ cup tomato paste
- 2 tablespoons butter
- 6 cloves of garlic, minced
- 2 teaspoons oregano
- ½ teaspoon crushed red pepper
- 1 pound cremini or white mushrooms, stems removed and quartered
- 1 (14 ounce) can diced tomatoes
- ½ cup chicken stock
- ½ cup dry red wine
- 3 pounds boneless, skinless chicken thighs
- Sea salt and pepper to taste

Instructions:

1. Combine the onions, tomato paste, butter, garlic, red pepper, and oregano in a microwave safe bowl. Microwave, on high, for 3-5 minutes. Stirring occasionally.
2. Add the mixture to your slow cooker and stir in the quartered mushrooms, diced tomatoes, chicken stock, and wine.
3. Season the chicken with salt and pepper and add to the slow cooker.
4. Cook for 4-6 hours on low.
5. Garnish with fresh basil, if desired.

Lemon Butter Roasted Chicken
Serves 6-8

Ingredients:

- 1 whole chicken, about 4-5 pounds, depending on the size of your slow cooker
- 1 cup chicken stock
- ½ teaspoon sea salt
- ½ teaspoon black pepper
- 1 whole lemon, sliced thinly
- 4 tablespoons butter
- 2 tablespoons fresh parsley

Instructions:

1. Pat your chicken dry and be sure to discard the giblets inside.
2. Season well with salt and pepper and place into your slow cooker.
3. Pour the stock into the bottom of the slow cooker.
4. Cook on high for 3 hours. Chicken is ready when it reaches an internal temperature of 165 degrees Fahrenheit.
5. Just before serving, melt the butter in a small saucepan. Add the lemon slices and simmer until the lemons darken in color.
6. Pour the mixture over the chicken and garnish with fresh parsley.
7. Serve!

Fajita Chicken
Serves 4-6

Ingredients:

- 2 pounds boneless, skinless chicken breasts
- 1 yellow onion, sliced
- 2 bell peppers, sliced
- 4 cloves of garlic, minced
- 1 teaspoon sea salt
- 1 teaspoon coriander
- 1 teaspoon oregano
- ½ teaspoon cumin
- ½ teaspoon chili powder
- 1 (14 ounce) can diced tomatoes
- Bib or leaf lettuce for serving

Instructions:

1. Lay chicken breasts in the bottom of your slow cooker.
2. Top with the sliced onions and peppers and garlic.
3. Sprinkle the seasonings on top then add the diced tomatoes. Do not stir.
4. Cook on low for 6 hours or high for 4 hours.
5. Once the chicken is cooked, shred with tongs or two forks.
6. Mix well and serve with lettuce to wrap the chicken.

Coconut-Lemongrass Chicken Drumsticks
Serves 5

Ingredients:

- 10 drumsticks, skin removed
- 1 tablespoon lemongrass paste
- 4 cloves of garlic
- 1 tablespoon fresh ginger, grated
- 1 cup coconut milk (canned)
- 2 tablespoons fish sauce
- 1 teaspoon Chinese five spice powder
- 1 yellow onion, thinly sliced
- Sea salt and pepper to taste

Instructions:

1. Season the chicken drumsticks generously with salt and pepper.
2. Add the sliced onion to the bottom of your slow cooker. Place the chicken on top.
3. In a blender or food processor, combine the remaining ingredients. Blend until well combined.
4. Pour mixture on top of the chicken and cook on low for 4-5 hours.
5. Garnish with sliced green onions, if desired.

Chile, Chicken & Lime Soup
Serves 5

Ingredients:

- 2 pounds boneless, skinless chicken breasts
- 2 tablespoons olive oil
- 1 (8 ounce) package of mushrooms, sliced
- 1 yellow onion, diced
- 1 tomato, diced
- 5 cloves of garlic, minced
- 1 (5 ounce) can diced green chilies
- 1/3 cup lime juice
- 6 cups chicken broth
- 1 teaspoon chili powder
- ½ teaspoon cumin
- ½ teaspoon oregano
- sea salt and pepper to taste
- Sliced avocado (garnish)
- Chopped cilantro (garnish)

Instructions:

1. Season the chicken with salt and pepper.
2. In a large skillet, over medium-high heat, cook the chicken until browned on both sides. Set aside to cool.
3. Place the remaining ingredients (except for the garnishes) into your slow cooker.
4. Chop the cooked chicken and add to the slow cooker.
5. Cook on low for 8 hours.
6. Ladle into bowls and top with sliced avocado and cilantro. Serve!

Mediterranean Stuffed Chicken Breasts
Serves 4

Ingredients:

- 4 boneless, skinless chicken breasts
- 1 tablespoon olive oil
- ½ red onion, diced
- ½ red bell pepper, thinly sliced
- 2 cups fresh baby spinach
- 1 clove garlic, minced
- 1 teaspoon dried oregano
- sea salt and pepper to taste
- juice of ½ a lemon
- 1 cup chicken stock
- ½ cup dry white wine
- fresh parsley, chopped (garnish)

Instructions:

1. Cut a deep slit in the side of each chicken breast, so that it forms a pocket. Season the chicken with salt and pepper.
2. Heat the olive oil in a large skillet over medium-high heat. Cook the peppers and onions and cook until softened. Add the garlic and spinach and cook until the spinach is wilted. Add the oregano and remove from heat and allow to cool.
3. Stuff each chicken breast with equal amounts of the spinach mixture.
4. Add the chicken breasts to your slow cooker and squeeze the lemon juice over the top.
5. Add the chicken stock and white wine to the slow cooker and cook on low for 6-8 hours or high for 4 hours.
6. Garnish with fresh parsley and serve.

Chicken Tikka Masala
Serves 6

Ingredients:

- 6 boneless, skinless chicken thighs
- 2 tablespoons olive oil
- 1 yellow onion, diced
- 2 cloves of garlic, minced
- 2 teaspoons sea salt
- 1 ½ tablespoons garam masala
- 1 teaspoon paprika
- 3 tablespoons tomato paste
- 1 (28 ounce) can diced tomatoes
- 1 (15 ounce) can coconut milk
- Cilantro (garnish)

Instructions:

1. Heat the olive oil in a large skillet over medium-high heat. Add the chicken and cook until browned on all sides. Transfer the chicken to your slow cooker.
2. Sauté the onion in the same pan as the chicken and cook until translucent. Add the garlic, salt, garam masala, and paprika. Stir to combine.
3. Stir in the tomato paste and diced tomatoes. Bring to a simmer. Remove from heat and stir in the coconut milk.
4. Pour the mixture over the chicken and cook for 6-8 hours on low or 4 hours on high, removing the lid to allow the sauce to thicken during the last half hour of cooking.
5. Garnish with fresh cilantro and serve.

Easy Balsamic Chicken
Serves 4

Ingredients:

- ½ cup balsamic vinegar
- ½ cup chicken stock
- ¼ cup honey
- 3 cloves of garlic, minced
- 4 bone-in, skin-on chicken breasts
- 1 teaspoon dried basil
- ½ teaspoon dried oregano
- ¼ teaspoon dried thyme
- ¼ teaspoon dried rosemary
- Sea salt and pepper
- Fresh parsley, chopped (garnish)

Instructions:

1. Season the chicken breasts with the spices and place in your slow cooker.
2. In a small bowl, whisk together the balsamic vinegar, chicken stock, honey, and garlic. Pour over the chicken.
3. Cook low for 7-8 hours or high for 3-4 hours. Chicken is ready when it reaches an internal temperature of 165 degrees Fahrenheit.
4. Serve immediately and garnish with fresh parsley.

Chicken Meatball and Veggie Soup
Serves 5-6

Ingredients:

- For the meatballs:
- 1 pound ground chicken
- 3 tablespoons Italian seasoning
- 2 tablespoons dried basil
- 2 tablespoons ground flax
- 1/3 cup white onion, grated

- For the soup:

- 4 cups chicken or vegetable stock
- 1 ½ cups water
- 2 (14.5 ounce) cans diced tomatoes
- 3-4 carrots, peeled and chopped
- 2 cups peas
- 3-4 celery stalks, chopped
- 2 cloves of garlic, minced

Instructions:

1. Place all of the ingredients for the vegetable soup into your slow cooker.
2. Cook on low for 3-4 hours.
3. Prepare the meatballs by combining all of the ingredients together. Mix well using your hands.
4. Roll into balls that are about 1" in size.
5. Place in the refrigerator until the soup has cooked for 3-4 hours.
6. Drop the meatballs into the soup and turn the slow cooker to high heat. Cook for about an hour, until they are cooked through.
7. Serve immediately.

Chicken Mole
Serves 5-6

Ingredients:

- 2 pounds chicken pieces (breasts and thighs work well)
- Sea salt and pepper
- 2 tablespoons coconut oil
- 1 yellow onion, diced
- 4 cloves of garlic, minced
- 1 (28 ounce) can whole, peeled tomatoes
- 5 dried chili peppers, rehydrated and chopped
- ¼ cup almond butter
- 3 squares dark chocolate (70% cocoa or above)
- 1 teaspoon cumin
- ½ teaspoon cinnamon
- ½ teaspoon chili powder
- Diced avocado (garnish)
- Chopped cilantro (garnish)

Instructions:

1. Season the chicken pieces generously with salt and pepper.
2. In a large skillet, over medium-high heat, melt the coconut oil. Add the chicken and cook until browned on all sides.
3. Transfer the chicken to your slow cooker.
4. Add the onion to pan used to cook the chicken and saute until translucent. Add the garlic and cook an additional 1-2 minutes. Transfer the onion and garlic to the slow cooker.
5. Add the tomatoes, chili peppers, almond butter, dark chocolate, and spices to the slow cooker.
6. Cook on low for 4-6 hours, until the chicken is tender and pulls apart easily.
7. Serve topped with avocado and fresh cilantro.

Simple Chicken Soup
Serves 4

Ingredients:

- 2 boneless, skinless chicken breasts
- 2 boneless skinless chicken thighs
- 1 medium onion, diced
- 3 celery stalks, diced
- 3 carrots, peeled and diced
- 1 teaspoon apple cider vinegar
- 1 tablespoon Italian seasoning
- 1 teaspoon sea salt
- ½ teaspoon black pepper
- 4 cups water

Instructions:

1. Add the vegetables to your slow cooker and place the chicken pieces on top.
2. Sprinkle the Italian seasoning, salt and pepper on top.
3. Pour in enough water to cover the vegetables and come about halfway up the chicken. (About 4-5 cups)
4. Cook on low for 6-8 hours.
5. Remove the chicken and allow to cool slightly. Shred the chicken and add back to the slow cooker. Adjust seasonings and add more water, if necessary.
6. Serve and enjoy!

Creamy Chicken and Kale Soup
Serves 6

Ingredients:

- 4 cups shredded chicken (a rotisserie chicken works great)
- 6 cups chicken stock
- 1 bunch kale
- 3 lemons
- 2 tablespoons lemon juice
- 1 yellow onion, diced
- ½ cup olive oil
- Salt and pepper to taste

Instructions:

1. Wash and cut the kale into ½" strips.
2. Add 2 cups of chicken stock, onions, and olive oil to your blender or food processor. Blend until smooth and creamy.
3. Transfer the mixture to your slow cooker and pour in the remaining stock.
4. Add the chicken, kale, lemon juice, and zest of the 3 lemons. Season with salt and pepper.
5. Cook on low for 6 hours, stirring once or twice.
6. Serve!

Honey-Garlic Chicken Wings
Serves 6

Ingredients:

- 2-3 pounds chicken wings
- 2 tablespoons olive oil
- 5-6 cloves of garlic, minced
- ¾ cup honey
- Sea salt and pepper to taste

Instructions:
1. Place the chicken wings into your slow cooker.
2. In a small bowl, mix together the remaining ingredients.
3. Pour over the chicken wings and cook for 6 hours on low or 3-4 hours on high.
4. Be careful not to overcook as you don't want the meat falling off the bones.
5. Enjoy!

Italian Style Chicken and Sausage
Serves 6-8

Ingredients:

- 4 boneless, skinless chicken breasts
  6 fresh Italian sausage links (sweet or spicy fine)
  1 white onion, thinly sliced
  4-6 cloves of garlic, minced
  Extra virgin olive oil
  1 teaspoon Italian seasoning
  1 teaspoon garlic powder
  1 teaspoon salt
  2 (14.5 ounce) cans diced tomatoes
  1 (15 ounce) can tomato sauce
  1 cup water or chicken stock
  1/2 cup balsamic vinegar
  1 teaspoon Italian seasoning
  1/2 teaspoon salt
  1/2 teaspoon garlic powder

Instructions:

1. Place the chicken breasts in the bottom of your slow cooker and sprinkle with the Italian seasoning, garlic powder, and salt.
2. Lay the sausage over the chicken and then the sliced onion and minced garlic.
3. Pour in the diced tomatoes, tomato sauce, chicken stock, and balsamic vinegar.
4. Sprinkle with the additional Italian seasoning, garlic powder and salt.
5. Cook on high for 5 hours.
6. Serve over spaghetti squash, zucchini noodles, or on it's own!

Kimchi Chicken
Serves 6

Ingredients:

- 2 pounds boneless, skinless chicken thighs
- 1 cup chicken stock
- 6 cloves of garlic, minced
- 1 tablespoon coconut aminos
- 2 teaspoons honey
- 1 tablespoon sesame oil
- 1 teaspoon fresh ginger, grated
- 2 cups kimchi
- 1 bunch green onions, sliced

Instructions:

1. Combine the chicken stock, garlic, coconut aminos, honey, sesame oil, and ginger in the bottom of your slow cooker. Give a good stir.
2. Nestle the chicken thighs into the sauce.
3. Cook for 4-6 hours on low.
4. When almost ready to serve, crank the heat to high and add the kimchi. Cook for an additional 20 minutes.
5. Garnish with sliced green onions and serve!

Tandoori Chicken
Serves 4-6

Ingredients:

- 2 pounds boneless, skinless chicken breasts
- 4 cups chicken stock
- ½ yellow onion, finely diced
- 2 cloves garlic, minced
- Pinch of sea salt

- For the sauce:
- ½ cup coconut milk (canned)
- 1 teaspoon smoked paprika
- 1 teaspoon sea salt
- 1 teaspoon cayenne pepper
- 1 teaspoon cumin
- 1 teaspoon turmeric
- 1 teaspoon black pepper

Instructions:

1. Place the chicken breasts in the bottom of your slow cooker.
2. Add the chicken stock, onion, garlic, and salt. Cook on low for 8 hours.
3. In a small bowl, whisk together the coconut milk with all of the spices.
4. About 30 minutes before serving, pull the chicken apart using tongs or two forks.
5. Stir in the sauce and mix well.
6. Allow to cook for about 20-30 minutes.
7. Serve immediately. Great for lettuce wraps!

Weeknight Chicken with Mushrooms and Onions
Serves 2

Ingredients:

- 2 bone-in, skin-on chicken breasts
- 1 (8 ounce) package mushrooms, sliced
- 1 large yellow onion, sliced
- 1 cup chicken stock
- 2 teaspoons thyme
- Sea salt and pepper to taste

Instructions:

1. Line the bottom of your slow cooker with the sliced onions.
2. Place the chicken breasts on top.
3. Top the chicken breasts with the sliced mushrooms.
4. Sprinkle the thyme, salt, and pepper in.
5. Pour in the chicken stock and cook for 6-8 hours on low.
6. Chicken is ready when it reaches an internal temperature of 165 degrees Fahrenheit.

Chicken Marinara with Zucchini Noodles
Serves 4

Ingredients:

- 1 whole chicken, about 3-4 pounds
- 1 yellow onion, sliced
- 1 ½ cups marinara sauce
- Sea salt and pepper to taste
- 4 medium zucchini
- ¼ cup fresh basil, chopped

Instructions:

1. Place the sliced onion in the bottom of your slow cooker.
2. Generously season the chicken with salt and pepper. Add to the slow cooker.
3. Pour in the marinara sauce.
4. Cook on low for 6-8 hours or high for 3-4 hours.
5. Once the chicken has cooked, set it aside to cool slightly.
6. In the meantime, spiralize your zucchini into noodles. Place the noodles in a colander and sprinkle with salt. Allow the noodles to sit for 5 minutes. Squeeze out any excess water.
7. Shred the meat from the chicken and return to the slow cooker.
8. Toss the fresh basil with the zucchini noodles.
9. To serve, lay a bed of zucchini noodles down and spoon the chicken onto the noodles. Enjoy!

Bacon Wrapped BBQ Chicken
Serves 4

Ingredients:

- 4 boneless, skinless chicken breasts
- 1 ½ cups barbeque sauce (homemade is best to avoid high sugar content)
- 2 tablespoons lemon juice
- 4 apples, peeled and chopped
- 1 yellow onion, diced
- 8 slices of bacon

Instructions:

1. Wrap each chicken breast in 2 slices of bacon.
2. Place the bacon wrapped chicken in the bottom of your slow cooker.
3. In a bowl, combine the apples, barbeque sauce, lemon juice, and onion. Mix well.
4. Pour the barbeque mixture over the chicken and cook on low for 6-8 hours.
5. To serve, plate one of the chicken breasts and spoon the apple/onion mixture on top.

I hope you have enjoyed making these recipes. Feel free to provide me a review on amazon with your thoughts.

Until next time,
-Monica Marie

www.ingramcontent.com/pod-product-compliance
Lightning Source LLC
Chambersburg PA
CBHW071312280526
45788CB00004B/1884